My Journey with Lupus

From the Beginning to Now

By

Sheronda S. Hayes-Williams

My Journey with Lupus
From the Beginning to Now
Copyright © 2013 Sheronda S. Hayes-Williams
Edited by Author Sheila S. Rowell

Dedication

I would like to dedicate this book to my children Brandy, Courtney, and Kameron. Thank you for always caring for me when I couldn't do for myself, love you.

I'd like to thank my cousin Sheila (Keyla) Owens-Rowell for editing this book and for all the love and support she has given me throughout this process of dealing with my illness.

My Journey with Lupus

From the Beginning to Now

By

Sheronda S. Hayes-Williams

1

Lupus

MANY PEOPLE OFTEN wonder what "Lupus" is and what does it do to the human body. Well, for those individuals who may still be confused about this condition, Lupus is a disorder of the body's natural defense system (Immune System). In a person that has Lupus, the immune system attacks various areas of the body (Autoimmune Disease). There are four different types of Lupus, and in some cases, there can be an overlap in the symptoms, and each can affect the body differently as follows:

<u>Systemic Lupus Erythematosus</u> – (SLE) can affect nearly every part of the body, including the skin, joints, lungs, heart, central nervous system, kidneys, and the blood. This is form of Lupus that I have.

<u>Discoid Lupus Erythematosus</u> – (also called Cutaneous Lupus) affects only the skin. Its main symptoms include crusty, scaling sores on the face, on the head, and in other areas of the body.

Drug induced Lupus Erythematosus – is bought on by certain prescription medications; it usually goes away once the medication is stopped.

Neonatal Lupus – is rare, but happens when a mother passes Lupus antibodies to her unborn baby. The newborn baby may develop a rash and/or other symptoms that can last for several months and then disappear.

Symptoms of Lupus:

Lupus can affect many parts of the body, including the joints, skin, kidneys, lungs, heart, nervous system, and blood vessels. The sign and symptoms of Lupus differ from person to person. The disease can range from mild to life-threating. Typical features of Lupus include:

- Butterfly-shaped rash over the face.
- Arthritis involving one or more joints.
- Kidney disease.
- Fever, weight loss, hair loss, fatigue.
- Poor circulation in the fingers and toes.
- Chest pain when taking deep breaths; Abdominal pain may also occur.
- Skin rash in areas exposed to the sun.
- Sores in the mouth and nose.

2

The Beginning of my journey with Lupus

IT WAS JUNE 1992, and I was one month pregnant with my son Kameron; I was also preparing to get married. I already had two children, Brandy and Courtney, and life up to this point was good. I had a normal pregnancy with signs of problems. I didn't gain a lot of weight with any of my children, so my body snapped back quickly into shape. I had Kameron in February, but in April of that same year, I had lost a lot of weight but I didn't think anything of it, but many people had begun to ask me if I was ill. I paid little attention to what others were thinking; soon after that, I began to gain my weight back and I assumed that all was back to normal.

In July, I went for a urine test for a job, the lab tech was an older black lady. Looking very concerned, the lady looked me directly in the eyes and said, "Baby, you have too much protein in your urine." She continued to look concerned and advised me to make an appointment with my regular doctor as soon as possible. I didn't know if that was good or bad, but she finally told me that it was not good.

My regular doctor sent me to the lab for a 24 hour urine specimen and also ordered several other tests. The results of my labs came back conclusive and that I had Lupus. My doctor sat down with me and my husband at the time and talked to us about the disease. Just to hear the word "disease" was scary enough. I had heard of Lupus from a Soap Opera years ago, but I still didn't know what it actually was. When the doctor explained about the various ways that Lupus could affect a person, I viewed as a death sentence. What I had learned soon after the results of my labs were complete regarding the Lupus is listed below:

- Fact: Urine Test
- The antinuclear antibody (ANA) test can show if your immune system is more likely to make the autoantibodies of Lupus, most people with Lupus test positive for ANA but a positive ANA does not mean you have Lupus. About five to ten percent of healthy women test positive for ANA.
- Diagnosis – Diagnosing Lupus can take a long time and is often difficult. An exam and an account of your symptoms and health problems are very

important. Blood tests are necessary, although there is no single test that can confirm or rule out Lupus. Additional blood tests, and sometimes a kidney or skin tissue sample (Biopsy) can help to confirm or rule out Lupus.

My doctor then sent me to the University of Michigan hospital for more testing. I went every three months to a specialist. I was taking 65 mgs of prednisone (Steroids) which made me eat more than usual; I was weighing 130 lbs. prior to taking steroids, and 189 after. My entire presence changed and I didn't even know how to walk with the weight I gained. My face was so fat and round, if I smiled you couldn't even see my eyes. It was like I had a fat suit on when I looked at myself in the mirror. Depression set in and it wasn't nice, all I wanted to do was eat and sleep. My self-esteem and my confidence was now where to be found. Everyone tried to make me feel good about myself and the more they talked to me the more depressed I got.

I was so depress, I felt like everyone was staring at me and wondering what was happening to me. I remember my dad (Vergil), stated, "You look nice with that weight," and I felt that he was just trying to make me feel better, but nothing anyone said actually worked. My husband had worked hard to make me feel special too, but I didn't. The disease was hard on the entire family. My husband felt helpless that he couldn't help me when I was in pain for there was nothing he could do; there was nothing no one could do. He would tell me that he would be right back but I didn't understand why he would leave me when I was in so much pain. Later on, I discovered that he was having a hard time seeing me like that and he hated the fact that he couldn't help me. His heart was heavy seeing me in pain.

Brandy, my eldest daughter, would cry an awful lot in school and no one knew what was going on with her. The teacher came to me one day and asked if there was anything unusual going on in the home. I had to tell her about my illness. I tried not to cry in front of the children but it was hard not to because I had been in so much pain. Some days, the pain would become so unbearable, especially during the mornings. In knowing more about my journey with Lupus, and learning about other individuals who are suffering from it, it has become very clear how this illness can affect the entire family, in many different ways.

On one of my scheduled doctor's appointments, I was informed by my family doctor to have my tube's tied. I had three children already but I wanted that to be a choice that I would make when and if I decided to have this procedure done; this was a personal situation that concerned my body, therefore, I wanted to have the right to decide for myself.

Eventually, I decided to have my tubes tied, and on the day of the surgery, I cried right up to the time that they put me under for the procedure. My mother (Faye) asks me why I was crying, and I just said I don't know. I also had to have a biopsy on my kidney; it was an overnight stay surgery procedure.

The doctor took three pieces of the kidney, he told me not to move while he was going through my back and as he continued with the procedure, I swear I could feel everything he was doing to me. I had to fight through this situation because in my mind, I knew that if I had moved, he could have punctured something else. I had to lay flat on my back until the next day. I had the biopsy done to check to see if the Lupus had affected my kidneys in anyway. That was a very scary procedure that I pray I never have to go through again.

Biopsy: Minor surgery to remove a sample of the tissue was performed. The tissue was then viewed under a microscope.

Finally, after going back and forth on the road for more labs and check-ups, I was able to locate a rheumatologist here in Muskegon, MI, so I stopped going to the hospital at the University of Michigan in Ann Arbor. Doctor Robert Hylland, the doctor that made it all clear to me, actually gave me the impression that he understood everything that I was going through, and somehow, just by him talking to me made me feel better. I thanked him for just listening to me; he was there through all of the rough times. I wasn't always the perfect patient either; I didn't like doing what I needed to do as far as getting my labs or taking medications that were prescribed to me. But, I had to face my issues and comply with the doctors' orders so that they could somehow improve my overall well-being.

Rheumatologist – a doctor that diagnose (detect) treat and medically manage patients with arthritis and other rheumatic diseases.

I become this mean nasty person, and people would say something about my weight and I would cry or cuss them out. My mother (Faye) would try to keep the conversation off of me if we were around other people. My mother asked the doctor to take me off the steroids or decrease the dosage because the medication was turning me into a very mean person and she wanted her mild-mannered daughter back. The doctor said that the steroids were making me aggressive but that he would taper my dosage down once the Lupus settled down. I began to hate the person I had become, and I would only shop at night so that I wouldn't have to run into people that I knew.

3

Cruelty & Misunderstand

PEOPLE CAN BE so cruel, especially when they don't know what's going on with you and why you look different. One of my classmates saw me in a store and told me that I looked like a pig; I thought that I would just die right where I was standing. I tried to explain to her that I was sick. She said, "You still don't have to eat so much!" I cried for days after that incident; her comment really broke me down. I prayed so hard every day for God to take this illness away from me.

My hair started falling out in spots, so I went to my beautician, (Sherri Briggs) and she said, "Let's just cut it down so it could hopefully grow back." I cried while she cut it and I think she did too. Sherri continued to talk to me the entire time, and told me that everything was going to be alright; this really made me feel good about getting it done. Sherri also told me about some hair pills that would help my hair grow back. She was one of my hero's during that time in my life, and I must admit, my hair was really cute after she had finished cutting and styling it.

There were many people that gave me positive words and thoughts, but among those people, other than my family, stood out more than others and provided me with the utmost support. This person actually took the time to research Lupus and actually taught me a thing or two about the disease that I was unaware of. That person is Mr. Michael Burt, and he has seen the good, the bad, and the ugly side of me, and instead of distancing himself from, we are still very close friends to this day. I just know that I appreciate him and I thank him for understanding me when no one else did, and I thank him for being there for me no matter what.

In order for family and friends to help and support you, they need to be educated and have some type of understanding about the disease. You have to let people know what to expect when the disease is active. God put a lot of people in my life to help me get through this disease and I want to do that for someone else.

I thought I was finally getting a hold on my Lupus condition, then the divorce happened; the stress from that really aggravated my Lupus. I had a flare up, a huge flare up. I had hair loss, weight loss, depression and fatigue. I didn't know if it was the Lupus or the fact that I was in a divorce, but it was a rough time period in my life. I tried to be private about the divorce but at the same time, I realized that by keeping things to myself and not even talking to my family about what was really going on with me didn't make it any better.

When I'm in pain, I try not to tell anyone because it seems like, in my mind anyway, people are saying, "What now!" There seems to always be something wrong but no one really wants to hear about it. That's when the happy face mask comes on, the one everyone sees, but on the inside, it was a whole different ballgame.

4

Using My Illness to Help Others

AFTER RECEIVING a call from one of my cousins who shared the devastating news of a relative being diagnosed with Lupus, she suggested that I pay her a visit and talk with her. I was terrified and I didn't want to talk to anyone about Lupus because I was still struggling with my own illness.

Lupus runs on my father's side of the family and many of them have more difficulty with it than I do. I didn't want to talk too much to them about it because I thought that by listening to their experience with Lupus, I felt that I wouldn't be able to handle it and the sadness of witnessing their personal struggles would overwhelm me. I look back at this event and see how silly I was for thinking this way, but that's the way I felt at the time.

After 19 years of being diagnosed with Lupus, I finally started researching the disease more in-depth; yes, it took several years for me to learn more about it. But, it took a very long while for me to face my fears, stop being angry, and live life as close to what I had been doing for so many years. I finally became more determined to not allow this illness to cripple me mentally because I can still engage in many activities that I have been doing for years, although I do have my painful moments, I am still alive.

As a cheerleading coach, you meet a lot of young ladies, and I have a squad of girls and during this particular year, I have had several flare ups with my Lupus. After a few days of my missing practice, the girls started calling me. I had to explain to the girls about my disease and what it does to me.

One of the girls went home and told her mom and the mother came to me the next day after practice wanting to speak with me. She told me that her daughter that was on my squad also had Lupus, but that her daughter was embarrassed to tell anyone. She also told me that her daughter thought that other children would pick on her or laugh at her because she had a disease. The mother asked me not to say anything to the child of what she had told me. I didn't understand why because I felt that I could have helped her understand what she was going through. I couldn't let it go, so what I did was talk about myself and my issues with the disease to the entire cheerleading squad.

Approximately 1 in 3 children with Lupus have mild disease, but most moderate disease that may be severe at times, but usually responds well to treatment. With proper diagnosis and treatment only a small number of children develop severe and life-threating Lupus.

5

My Journey with Lupus

MY MISSION IS to educate and to bring awareness about this chronic disease. It took me awhile to learn and understand how to cope with Lupus. I want to make it easy for someone else to understand and deal with it if I can.

I read about a Lupus Walk and wanted to attend it, but I missed it because it was held in Chicago. I decided to have one in my home town (Muskegon, Michigan). I was very proud to do that although it was a lot of work, more than I had bargained for. Getting the sponsors and the materials together it was work. The Walk for Lupus was on May 11, 2013 at the Muskegon Heights High School and half of the proceeds were to go to the Lupus Foundation of America for research and a cure, the other half to the Muskegon Health Project. Unfortunately the walk was rained out, and all my hard work went down the drain, or so I thought. All the advertisement I had done for the Walk brought awareness to the community.

People would see me and ask me what is Lupus, or they would tell me about someone in their family that had

Lupus. I would also receive calls from other Lupus patients that asked questions such as, "Do you have this kind of pain," or "What do you do to relieve pain?" The walk regarding Lupus presented a multitude of information for individuals who had little to no idea about what Lupus is. Although the rain prevented a much larger turn out, those who did show up made the event well worth it. I plan to have other walks and events regarding Lupus in the future.

6

Living, Loving, & Learning with Lupus

WHILE WORKING at a local grocery store, the first boss I had already knew about Lupus. My boss had gotten to the point where he knew exactly when I was having a flare up just by looking at me and he was very sympathetic. Three years later I got another boss same work place, I told him about Lupus and gave him some literature on it and he was also sympathetic. But, then I got another boss, at the same job, that didn't care about what I had, he was more concerned about his motto, "Just get the job done." The lesson here is to understand that regardless of who you are or what type of illness you might have, everyone will not is not going to be as caring or sympathetic as some people.

My journey with Lupus has strengthened my faith in God, and it has truly educated my family and close friends about the disease. Although both of my adult daughter have tested positive for Lupus, their journey is still fresh and new, but unlike myself, they have yet to be further tested and provided with treatment; my condition seemed to come out in full bloom once I learned about it. I will always be there for my daughters and together, our journey with Lupus will give us the energy to reach out to others who may have the disease or who may know someone else that does. I will continue making an effort to learn more about Lupus, regardless of how it affects me, my ongoing goal is to find ways to reach out to others and offer as much assistance as possible so that more people can understand how Lupus can affect others, because the more we know, the more we can grow and develop ways to reach out to others, because by extending our hand out to them, they can eventually do the same for someone else.

Nonetheless, I may have Lupus, but Lupus does not have me, for I am a survivor and a fighter. Just like the butterfly, I will continue to soar freely while holding my head up high, and graciously move with the wind and continue on my journey, living my life with Lupus.

My advice for anyone who is suffering from Lupus, and/or anyone who has a family member or friend that has Lupus:

- ✓ Be supportive
- ✓ Educate yourself
- ✓ If you are an immediate family member, get tested

✓ Motive, Inspire, and continue to learn more about Lupus so that you will understand at least the basics about the disease and how it may affect someone

Share your daily thoughts about whatever illness or illnesses, that you struggle or someone close to you are dealing with on the following pages………..

Daily Words, Thoughts, and Phrases

Daily Words, Thoughts, and Phrases

Daily Words, Thoughts, and Phrases

Daily Words, Thoughts, and Phrases

Daily Words, Thoughts, and Phrases

Daily Words, Thoughts, and Phrases

Daily Words, Thoughts, and Phrases

Daily Words, Thoughts, and Phrases

Daily Words, Thoughts, and Phrases

Daily Words, Thoughts, and Phrases

Daily Words, Thoughts, and Phrases

Daily Words, Thoughts, and Phrases

Daily Words, Thoughts, and Phrases

Daily Words, Thoughts, and Phrases

Daily Words, Thoughts, and Phrases

Daily Words, Thoughts, and Phrases

Daily Words, Thoughts, and Phrases

Daily Words, Thoughts, and Phrases

Daily Words, Thoughts, and Phrases

Daily Words, Thoughts, and Phrases

Daily Words, Thoughts, and Phrases

Daily Words, Thoughts, and Phrases

Daily Words, Thoughts, and Phrases

Daily Words, Thoughts, and Phrases

Daily Words, Thoughts, and Phrases

Daily Words, Thoughts, and Phrases

Daily Words, Thoughts, and Phrases

Daily Words, Thoughts, and Phrases

Daily Words, Thoughts, and Phrases

www.ingramcontent.com/pod-product-compliance
Lightning Source LLC
Chambersburg PA
CBHW070825290526
45795CB00002B/842